The Much
Calmer Sutra

The Much Calmer Sutra

RICHARD HUTT

NEW HOLLAND

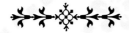
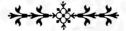
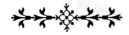
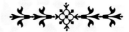
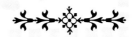

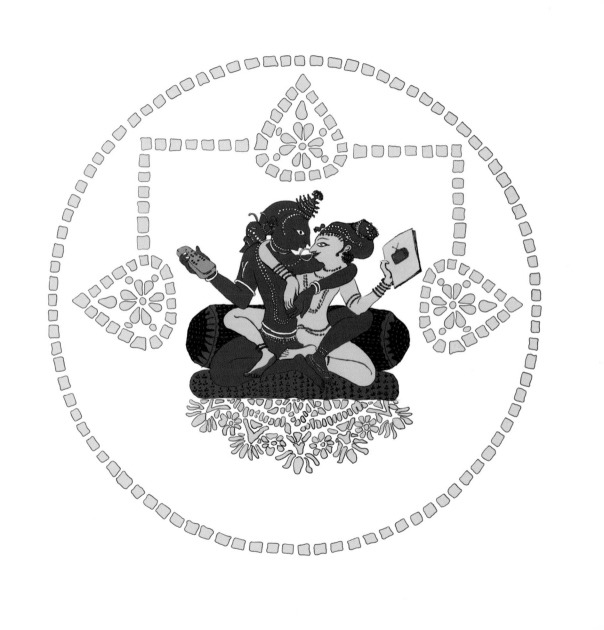

Introduction

The Much Calmer Sutra is a deceptively simple work. To the modern translator it might appear, at first glance, to state the obvious: namely that lying around with a loved one can be very pleasant indeed.

But it is in this very simplicity, this obviousness, that *The Much Calmer Sutra* shines brightest. In asking us to perform familiar, everyday acts with deliberate attention to detail, *The MCS* requires us to consider such "commonplace" pleasures as priceless jewels to be treasured. No longer should we take for granted those leisurely pursuits, those daily delights in which we so often forget to revel.

For the couple, this revelry serves a dual purpose. As we luxuriate in familiar pleasures, we may also take time to consider a wide array of relationship dynamics. Many of the positions illustrated herein afford us just such an opportunity – the chance to spend "quality time" in close quarters with our partner. It is time increasingly rare in the modern age and *The MCS* gives us many tools with which we may make the most of it.

One such tool is the model of the game. Several of these poses take the form of a contest, a battle of wills. In these it should be remembered that in many cases, the "victor" of a game may in fact "lose" in relationship terms. As one famed Sultan of the 10th century was heard to demur, following the loss of his prized peacock to a courtesan in such a game of chance: "no-one likes a winner."

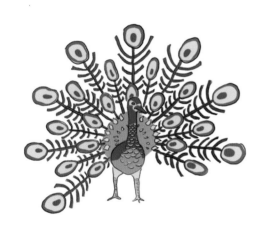

Although it may no longer literally cost us our heads to so triumph, we would do well to heed this advice, for as the scimitar of

that ancient monarch proves, none can make us suffer as dearly or as keenly as those closest to us.

It is a truism familiar to all who must share a bed, or a sofa, where the vengeance of a slighted partner may take many forms and cause us to rue our wrongs bitterly. Many such variations are, in fact, legitimate poses under the umbrella of *The Much Calmer Sutra* and they are featured here in the spirit of authenticity.

Other positions herein are more akin to a performance, in which each must play a part. Again, many couples may be tempted to bring emotional issues to these poses – this is to be expected and so he should not

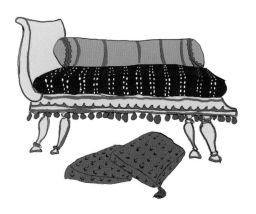

The History and Origins of MCS

The origins of *The Much Calmer Sutra* are obscure, vague and little understood. Certainly, the precepts that underpin the work pre-date that more famous cousin, the Kama Sutra. Cave-drawings as early as the Bronze Age clearly show gaily-dressed figures sporting themselves in a manner which might only be described as "louche".

Whatever the specifics of its origins, we do know that the delights of *The MCS* have been celebrated in many ancient societies. Many leisure cultures (those which have enjoyed a good amount of free time and the pleasures which a lack of manual labour make possible) show documentary evidence of a desire to lie about creatively.

express surprise should her anger rise on seeing him, say, take the prized position on the sofa – yet again. Rather let him enjoy the position and any accompanying "issues" or lengthy, heated discussions as a natural result of their love.

Thus Ancient Greece, Rome, India, the Far East – each have their own equivalent to the central text of *The Much Calmer Sutra*.

This was a world before Television. To understand *The MCS* in context, we must picture such a world, one in which "anything went" in the name of comfort, in which the long hours of the evening were to be filled with whatever forms of comfort should be deemed most satisfying.

The Inner Urge for Calm

That *The MCS* pre-dates the Kama Sutra should not be a surprise, for it answers a need that is stronger than any other human urge, a desire that we are all born with – the need to sit down. Indeed, some

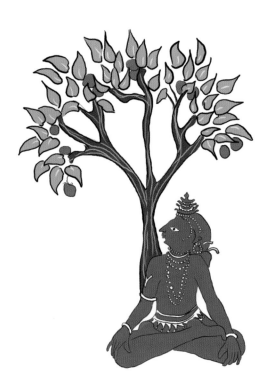

suggest that the very first position occurred when our ancestors chose to climb from the trees and assume a seated pose.

Other scholars, more radical still, point to instances of applied relaxation in the animal kingdom – e.g. the cat nap – and suggest that *The Much Calmer Sutra* brings us back to a primal joy which we lost the moment we came down from the trees, or crawled onto the shores.

The theory of "inherited memory" helps to explain why many of these poses may appear familiar to those who are studying *The MCS* for the first time. Indeed, some couples may be adapting the positions already without being aware they are simply "acting out" the patterns set by their forbears. A casual leaf through this translation may even cause some to cry out, seeing themselves in the illustrations, saying "Ha! This is you, my love, see, possessing the duvet, while I am represented by this person here, out in the cold."

While such guileless, unaware practice is not in itself necessarily unhealthy, regular indulgence without the use of a guide such as this may prove less than productive – and performing many poses unaided does risk accident.

The MCS and Modern Society

We may find it harder to justify now that we are wearing trousers, but the innate

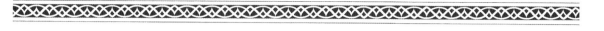

need for comfort is born within us. Society may laud the merits of hard work over pleasure, yet our inner animal cries out for satisfaction and will not rest until we rest.

It is a great irony that modern society, whilst denying the life-giving benefits of such systems, provides us with the tools by which we may enjoy them. With the discovery of fire, we may have lost the need to lie together – but fire begat central heating, which allows us all to attempt positions designed for temperate climates in the comfort of our own underwear.

Thus this book suggests poses by which the most profound and ancient of inner urges may be sated, with means readily available in the modern home, and so may we marshal the new in service of our true ancient desires.

A Word on Translation

What is most striking about *The MCS* is its continued relevance to our modern world. The parallels between the figures represented in ancient texts and the contemporary couple are striking. In place of the "sweetmeats" and "berry juice" of the original texts, we may have our "chocolate biscuits" and "tea", but the same principles inevitably apply. Similarly our modern beer may be substituted for the fermented juices of the Ancient World and household soap stand in for the perfumed unguents and coal tar of our forefathers.

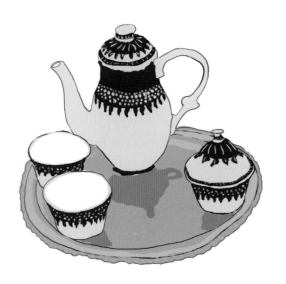

It must be stated that this is not a literal translation of a single text, rather a re-versioning of various ancient truths for a modern audience. Positions have on occasion been retitled to resonate with contemporary concerns. These texts have long been ignored and suppressed, reserved exclusively for the eyes of academics and students, willing to pore through ancient, forgotten tomes in dusty libraries. Hence only a few of these positions are public knowledge, for they have not been made truly accessible to a wider audience until now.

In fact, *The Much Calmer Sutra* has seen many translations and many interpretations, each of which says much about the society which begat them. A 17th century German text, for instance, saw the work as an invitation to labour and toil, whilst more recent Dutch versions have suggested a more… suggestive implication to the poses. Both must be taken with a healthy grain of salt. Ultimately, *The Much Calmer Sutra* is a broad body of work, lacking precise definition and drawing from a wide range of historical documents, folk art and hearsay.

These pages, then, are an editing, or "re-mix" of various sources, many of which must remain secret for reasons that space precludes us from detailing here, but which are eminently sensible. The keen reader will be assured to learn that such

sources offer material fit for many, many more volumes.

The Positions and a Word on Safety

The positions that follow are modern re-enactments of ancient ones, with illustrative contexts which suggest where they might take place. The text that accompanies each position gives background to the pose – its history, meaning and relevance – as well as tips on how to best perform it and guidance on relationship issues that may result from its use.

There are many types of position in *The Much Calmer Sutra*. For ease of use they are organised here into the areas of the home in which they may take place. The many emotional sub-texts apparent in each offer another approach, for some may choose to perform them following his or her own feelings – when, for instance, the other partner wishes to atone for alleged misdeeds.

In all cases, couples are advised to take each position step-by-step. Do not rush to the most complex first, though the temptation may be strong. Learn to sit before you attempt to lie.

In Conclusion: The Finding of True Calm

Were we ever more in need of a textbook to relationship happiness than now? Faced with the thousand demands of the modern world, we rarely take the time to enjoy simply "being" with our loved ones and traditional poses may be taken without thought, thus without the return of pleasure. We have, in essence, forgotten how to celebrate both our differences – and indifferences. This work humbly seeks to return them to us.

In following *The Much Calmer Sutra*, the modern couple is embarking on a journey for which these positions are but a starting point. Such a journey may seem familiar, for an ancient urge underpins all such poses, an innate knowledge of the true path to happiness. The body knows its own

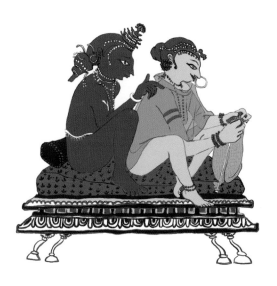

joys better than the mind and so there is a chance that in the process of enacting the positions, the couple may find a variation, which is of significantly greater pleasure for both.

This book not only notes, but actively encourages all such variations. For the rules of *The Much Calmer Sutra* only apply as long as the practitioners seek guidance and when the desire for comfort is strong, all other rules must fall away. For there is one eternal truth which towers above all positions – relaxation and comfort must find their own path. Or, as one ancient, and anonymous, sage put it: "If it feels good, do it."

The Sofa

The sofa is the true spiritual home of *The Much Calmer Sutra*. For here are our relationship battles played out, over fields of cushions. Here does compromise comfort make, and selfishness beget rancour. Many are the couples whose happiness has been sacrificed over unfairly distributed sofa acreage.

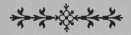

In the modern age, various props accompany our use of the sofa: chief among them are the television and its all-important symbol of power, the remote control. Many positions suggest a means by which this power may be shared – however, some scholars suggest that every partnership must by definition contain one "controller" and one "controlled", who must yield to the other's choices regarding entertainment. In such cases, for reasons of balance, it is recommended that the roles here are reversed and that s/he who is most accustomed to control may experience a lack thereof. Cushions, like nudity, are considered optional yet desirable, adding exciting variants for the positions that follow.

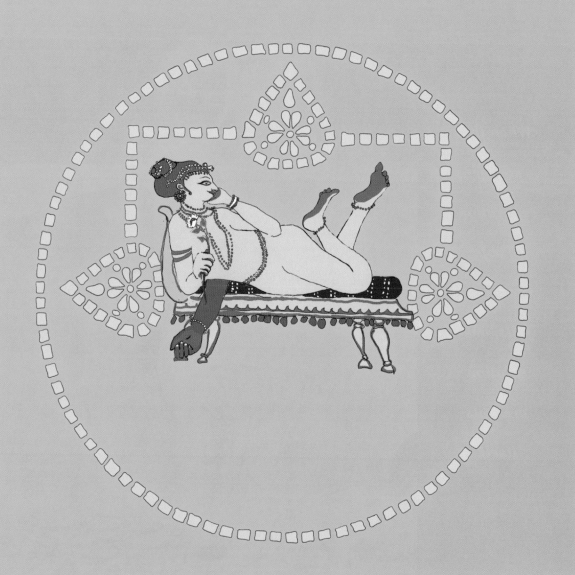

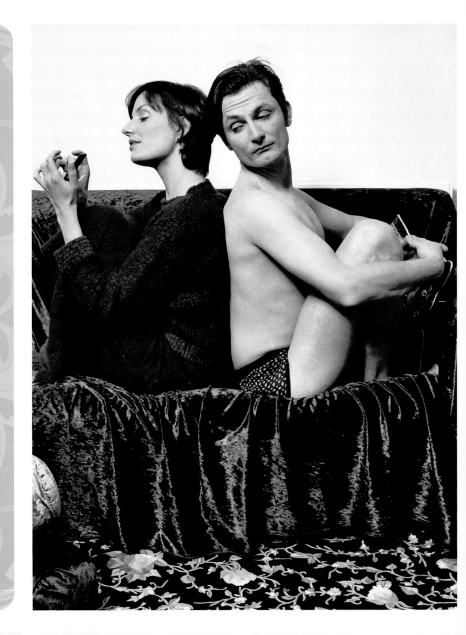

When the ad-hoc separation of sofa acreage fails, one solution presents itself.

Bookends

Many positions herein allow partners a liberal approach to space, an opportunity to divide the cushion area as appropriate and according to mood. While some couples can trust each other to respect mutual boundaries and take only the space they need, others may find that certain relationship issues raise their heads here, leading to a selfish grabbing for land.

"Bookends" allows the couple to recapture any lost feelings of trust, while ensuring an equal distribution of seating. Each sits in the centre of the sofa. At a given sign, both turn and swivel feet upwards (having first ensured that footwear is removed.) The backs now press against each other. Both bring their knees towards the chest. In this manner do they then relax, taking in their hands periodicals of the day, word-games, puzzles and the like.

A cushion may be slipped in-between the two seated partners for additional comfort.

Should such entertainments fail to amuse, one may then turn to the other in search of alternative pastimes. Such distractions from the matter at hand may prove unwelcome and risk pains in the area of the neck.

99 and a Half

This position, amongst the oldest in the world, arose among the servant classes of ancient Assyria. These unlucky souls were forced to make bed as best they could, amongst the corridors and mezzanines of the splendid palaces in which they toiled. The craft and ingenuity which they employed is here updated for contemporary spaces of limited comfort, such as self-assembly sofas of Swedish origin and the spare bedrooms of distant relatives.

Let the first partner lie on their side, forming the shape of the numeral "9", lacing the fingers of both hands behind the neck and curling the back while extending both feet, knees together and toes pointed. The other partner should then settle immediately in front of the first and set to mimicking the move, in close proximity. The nose of the partner behind may be brought to touch the nape of the neck of the other. The upper arm of the former should then be laid lengthways behind the latter, if possible grasping or "cupping" the buttock. This act is the additional "half" of the title.

However, special attention must be paid to the proximity of the gluteal area to the regions of the groin of the partner behind, who, finding their field of vision limited, is likely to seek some form of physical amusement. Ancient Assyria held such behaviour to invite unwelcome and unhealthy distraction from spiritually "pure" relaxation and those so cavorting were liable to face long careers as Eunuchs.

Comfort requires sacrifice: he who commands soft cushions may pay some other way.

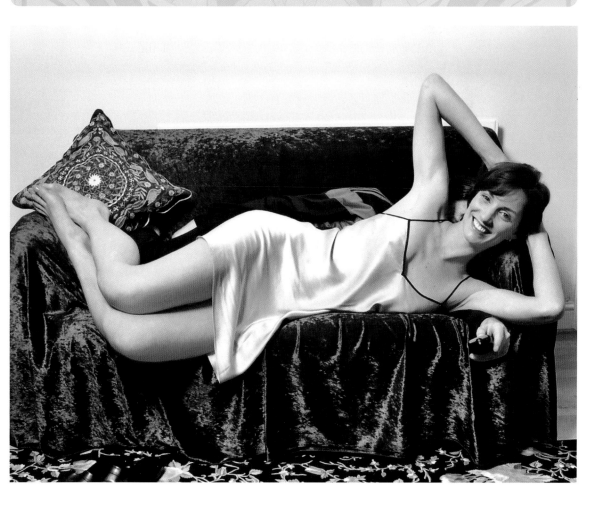

Thus recumbant, he or she may delight in their new status as "monarch" of the sofa.

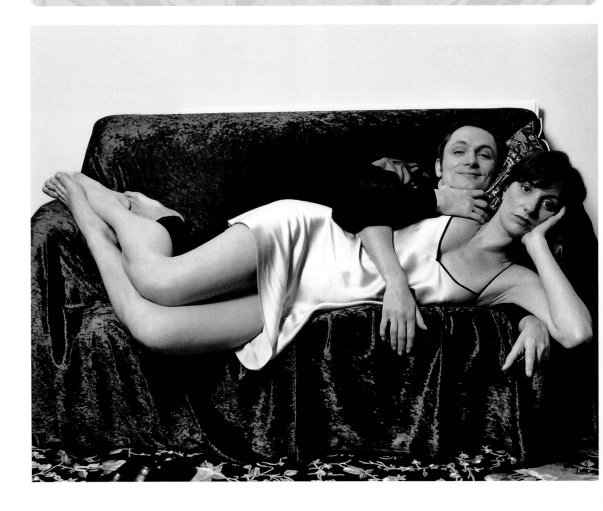

The 100

"The 100" is an expanded, "deluxe" version of the classic "99 and a Half".
While offering supreme comfort in limited circumstances, "99 and a Half"
has one primary drawback – it is not suitable for the simultaneous
enjoyment of visual stimulation. Hence the position know as "The 100",
in which our ancestors employed small livestock to cushion and raise
the head, thus allowing two partners to enjoy spectator sports and
ritual theatrical dramas in mutual comfort.

Most contemporary scholars agree that an actual cushion is an
acceptable modern substitute for livestock. The pygmy goat, while
offering an authentic experience (and an excellent pet), may simply
mean far too much effort for today's modern couple, pressed for time.

Assume the position of the "99 and a Half" as illustrated on the preceding
page. Let the partner behind the forward partner position one pillow/goat
between ear and sofa. Tilting the head, as if a coy teenager, let them
then use the upper arm to pull the front partner towards and down,
allowing a clear line of sight to any visual spectacle presented nearby. Thus
recumbant, he or she may delight in their new status as "monarch" of the
sofa. Be warned, though, that the question of desirable entertainment
does now become an issue.

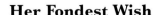

Her Fondest Wish

As the position, "His Prerogative", later shows, we may all benefit from the studied application of personal indulgence. Some occasions call for this in particular: and many women may find this position of comfort during their monthly responsibilities.

Let her recline at length, taking full command of sofa and, grumbling, let her dictate his position, demanding he go this way and that. Finally he may be ordered to rest, seated, under her extended feet. Taking her feet in his hands let him then do as she bids, rubbing this way and that and speaking words that are agreeable to her, such as "that's right" and "oh yes, my dear?"

She may then choose to bid him to fetch sweetened treats, chocolates and the like, and to feed them to her, should they be deemed satisfactory.

In this way may women be placated and soothed, but folly on the man who takes such indulgence to mean he is gifted with forgiveness. For no man may be truly forgiven during this period and should instead wish only to be forgotten briefly.

For no man may be truly forgiven during this period and should instead wish only to be forgotten briefly.

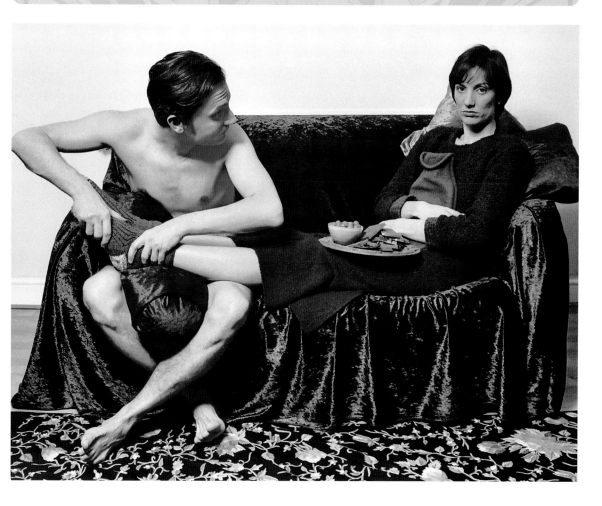

Thus offering the flesh as pillow, one partner earns the right do as they will, free from interruption.

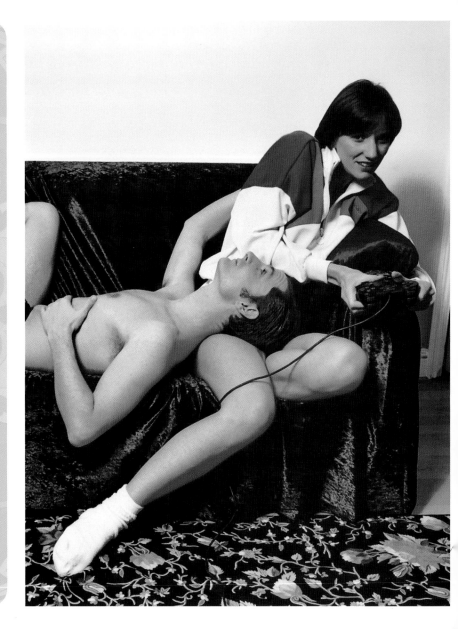

The Pillow

In the position "The Final Lap" we will see how noble self-sacrifice can benefit both parties. By assuming the form of comfort object we accrue in return Karmic credit, or "comfort tokens" which we may later choose to redeem at our leisure, saying "I have helped you, and now it is your turn to do likewise." In "The Pillow" the debt is repaid immediately.

Let one assume a seated position of comfort at the far end of the sofa, and take up such entertainments as are offered. Let the other now lower the head, nestling it on the thighs of the seated party. Gentlemen may especially care to exercise caution when positioning the recumbent head around the groinal regions. In such a position, the prostrate partner has little to entertain them save the countenance of the other, while the Pillow has a wider range of pleasures available.

A word of caution: both sexes should note that this position renders the protection offered by "Silent but Deadly" utterly ineffective. Hence trust here is vital and he (or she) who violates it may endure terrible punishments.

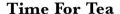

Time For Tea
(Or: a treatise on the correct means of exchanging fluids.)

Along with various comforts, partnership confers on each lover important responsibilities. The greatest of these is the fetching of hot brewed beverages. Reclining, each partner should seek to elect the other as responsible for the duties associated with the task. He should entreat her, making reference to the hardships of the working day, whilst she may refer to physical ailments or other impediments. Both should speak of recent duties discharged, such as the preparation of foodstuffs.

That partner who relents first is nominated to be the one responsible for preparation of the tea. This honour also falls on anyone who should happen to be standing when beverages are first mentioned.

Having prepared the beverages according to manufacturer's instructions, the partner must then exercise gentle caution in delivering it to their recumbent lover. The full vessel should be placed directly, handle first, into the hand, without having spilled a drop. If placing on floor or table, the partner must correctly adjudge the distance between drinker and drink, and shall not place it further than the radius of the outstretched hand, for this is an act of pronounced cruelty. Even when the ceremony is enacted as described here, yet the seated one may express displeasure, saying "Sit down; you have blocked my field of vision." For some people are never happy.

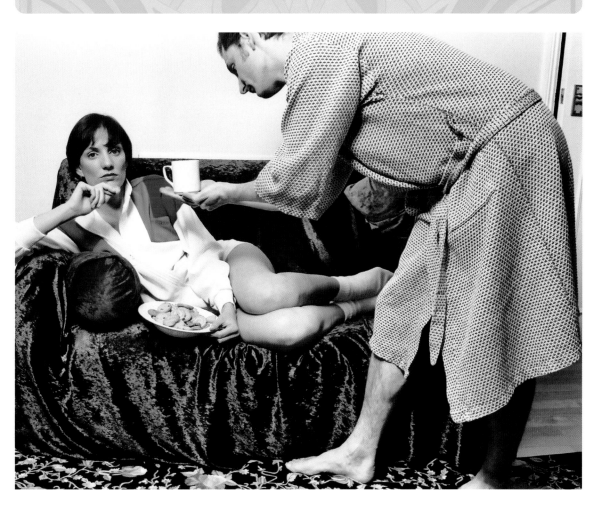

Along with various comforts, partnership confers on each lover important responsibilities.

A perfect demonstration of that central Much Calmer Sutra axiom, "Two can live more comfortably than one".

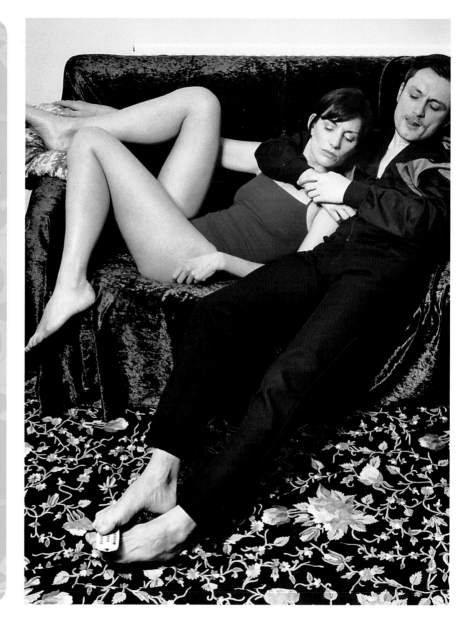

Dipping the Toe

Man is driven by two conflicting impulses: the drive to make his mark on the world; and his deep-seated need to do as little as possible, as much of the time as possible. *The Much Calmer Sutra* teaches a middle path – a way that these two opposing forces may work together towards a full, rich, sedentary life. In this position, we also see how a couple harmoniously seek together towards mutual satisfaction with the active partner literally "stretching" themselves, so that what first appears to be a purely "lazy" act is proven in fact to work for the benefit of all.

Let the partner elected "controller" slide gently, in the prostrate position, from the sofa, *whilst remaining in constant physical contact with cushion*. The other partner or "Sack" may assist in support of this movement, providing a counter-balance which will serve to "anchor" the controller – for it is vital that they do not entirely part company, or the bonds of the position will be broken.

As they slide, they will send a single toe arcing towards whatever control mechanisms exist locally: television; light switch; magazines, etc., thus attempting to control that which surrounds them, without leaving the sanctity of the sofa. A perfect demonstration of that central Much Calmer Sutra axiom, "Two can live more comfortably than one".

His Prerogative

Though true partnership seeks equality in all things, yet *The Much Calmer Sutra* teaches us that certain positions need a particularly delicate balance between needs and requirements.

Let the more masculine of the partners (henceforth known as "he") assume control over the sofa by means of entreaties, trickery and gifts. His command of any controlling devices should now be expressed, to her chagrin, and in selecting entertainments, his choice should be that which is of no interest to her.

Sighing, let her turn away, and by means of physical innuendo, brewed barley beverages and attempted conversation seek to take his attention. In failing she must then re-double her efforts to converse, citing events of interest including local gossip, such as her views regarding the marriage prospects of distant friends. She may even choose to come to him dressed in fine silks and speak words of love but none such temptations may move he who is at one with his seating arrangements. Lastly let her sink into repose and seek solace in discussions of his merits with her family and friends. Beware, though, that ultimately the male partner may be invited, at her request, to consider such thoughts in a period of reflection overnight upon the sofa.

Such a position can assist in bringing the various issues of a relationship to light.

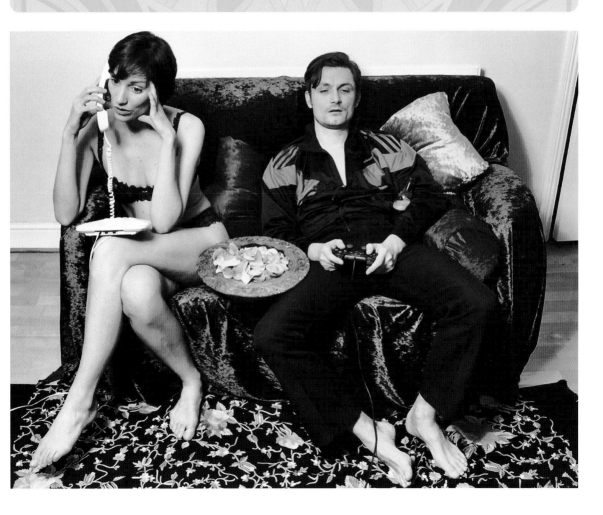

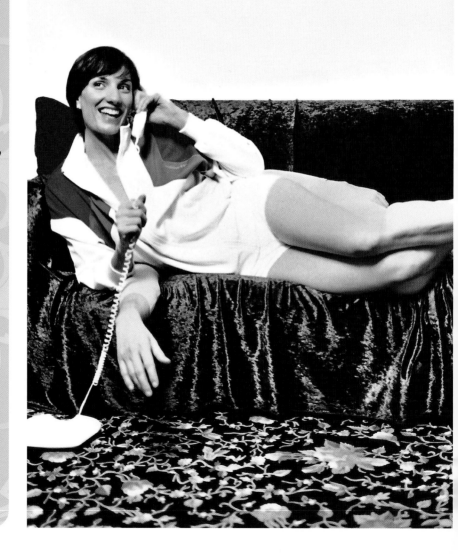

Some couples, over-familiar with each other's company, may find that the sofa is no longer the place of comfort and excitement it was in their earlier days.

Old Dead Arm

Some couples, over-familiar with each other's company, may find that the sofa is no longer the place of comfort and excitement it was in their earlier days. *The Much Calmer Sutra* suggests a very different approach: there can be, for the arms and legs of the dedicated seeker, life after death. With this position we learn to embrace the sensation of "pins and needles" as we embrace our loved one.

Let each lie according to their need side by side, his arm around her, underneath. He may slide his arm in the gap between her torso and lower arm to maximise the effect or may simply proffer it as pillow (this variation is known as the "Ultimate Sacrifice", for the limb utterly "dies" that his partner may live in comfort.)

He must then abide with the position until such time as she decrees to move. With stillness and bodily pressure may come unwelcome sensations, or even a lack thereof. He should breathe through these feelings and let his body relax, finding inspiration in the numbness. At no point must he refer, in words or sounds, to that pressure, or particularly to the bodily weight which may be behind it, for such comments may not be taken in a spirit of good humour.

The Final Lap

One may take his joy while the other toils and the correct balance of such acts is the most important part of their union. This is especially true in the modern relationship, in which restrictions of time, space and television may require that one of the two sacrifice their comfort in the short term, towards the long term happiness of both.

When one assumes the position of the chair, and the other of the sitter, then this is called "The Final Lap." Let the first person (typically the one who has rested whilst the other has toiled) sit, in chair or sofa, and take the part of the furniture, holding the legs still and straight at an angle of 90 degrees. The second partner then comes, and breathing out with the sound of "aaah" lowers themselves into the lap of the seated one.

Great care must be taken in the seating, particularly where the part of the chair is taken by the man. She must be cautious in her squirming, lest he cry out in pain, believing his reproductive capabilities to be threatened.

In this position we "become" furniture, proof of the transformative power of love and the nobility of sacrifice. The softness of flesh stimulates the central relaxation centre of the brain and promotes feelings of well-being. Such a compromise is particularly well suited to armchairs, rigid upright chairs, or situations where the entertainment needs of each partner may differ.

One may take his joy while the other toils.

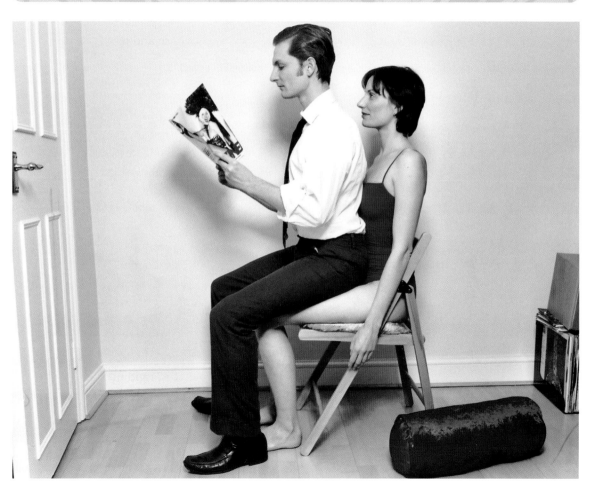

The Bed

Most of mankind's most basic, most primal desires are met in bed: sleep; warmth; food; television; and late night discussions of complex relationship issues.

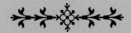

For any couple to be truly happy there must be a mutual and frank expression of bed-based needs. Lovers must be able to talk freely about the things that excite or please them; whether it be the cool side of the pillow or that side of the bed nearest the door. There may be some aspects of mutual bed-residence that she may find distasteful in him, or he in her – the thoughtless wandering of cold feet over warm flesh, for instance, or the production of noxious odours, similarly the stuffed animals and suchlike of childhood may also cause rancour – but only by confronting and defeating these issues can we learn to live a full and rewarding bed-life.

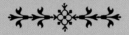

The positions that follow offer exciting starting points for couples who want to explore the possibilities offered by this stage of silk and cotton. Performing them will challenge both partners to stretch themselves and bring spice to their lying-down-time. The real secret to a satisfying bed-life is straightforward: a combination of communication, trust and high standards of personal hygiene.

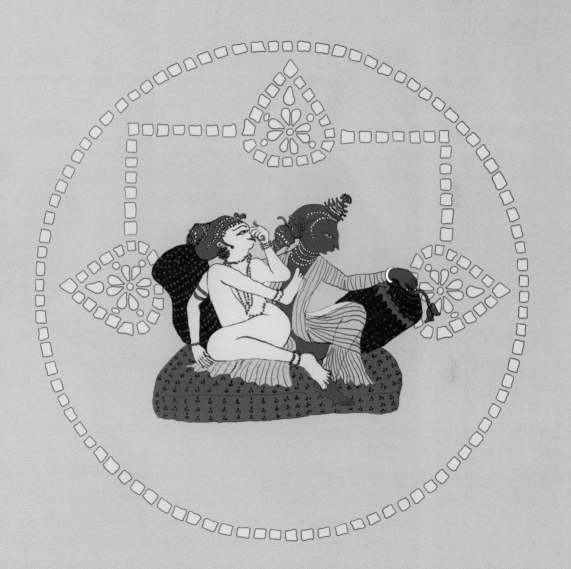

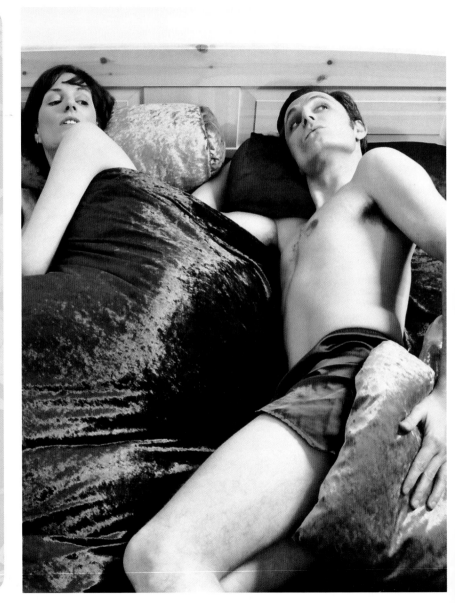

Unpleasantness should be avoided at all times and nowhere is this more true than in the confines of bed.

Silent, But Deadly

Lovers must seek always to shower their partner with the many wonderful fruits of life, sharing with them beautiful sights, sweet music and delightful smells. For the bed is a holy place, of great responsibility, and both should strive to keep this temple honourable and clean.

There may, however, be occasions upon which a partner will be faced with awkward decisions regarding the passing of noxious fumes. This position shows a means by which the responsible partner or "dealer" may take steps to protect the loved one from any odour which may be deemed less than savoury. This is particularly the case in the early weeks of their union, when both will be at pains to appear delightful to the other.

On first sign of internal distress, let him by his actions show nothing to be wrong, but under cover of conversation reach out for pillow or cushion and draw it to him. Let him position it as shown, push the posterior area with vigour towards it and, in so doing, let it envelop his undercarriage. Only then may he release his tightened muscles, remaining in this position until such time as it is deemed appropriate and any risk negligible.

Tradition has taught this act as the province of men, but powerful research, long suppressed, suggests that it may in truth be of equal use to both genders, strenuous denial notwithstanding.

Dances With Duvet

Love presents a struggle for power between the lovers, an eternal battle for control. "Dances with Duvet" offers the couple the chance to play out that struggle with high stakes: comfort; warmth; and ultimately… command of the bed.

Let each partner lie together and be draped with a covering of cotton, stuffed with the finest down. Let each after their own fashion make the sounds of sleep: yawning and stretching. Under cover of noise, taking a section of quilt in hand, let them grasp firmly. They will each then turn sharply and with strength and firm swift movement, attempt to envelop themselves in the covering, in the manner of the caterpillar, or the sausage which is wrapped in pastry.

The victor is he or she whose grip is strongest and who finds themselves in full command of the covering. The entreaties of the partner now left exposed shall include verbal pleadings and extravagant love promises, yet none of these shall move the comfortable partner to mercy. This position may also be enacted as a punishment by one partner, whilst the other delays in returning to the comfort of bed. Those who find this unjust may wish to consider the following ancient maxim: "the bed of the Princess is reserved for the punctual, while he who tarries upon the tiles is lucky to have any bed at all".

The bed of the Princess is reserved for the punctual, while he who tarries upon the tiles is lucky to have any bed at all.

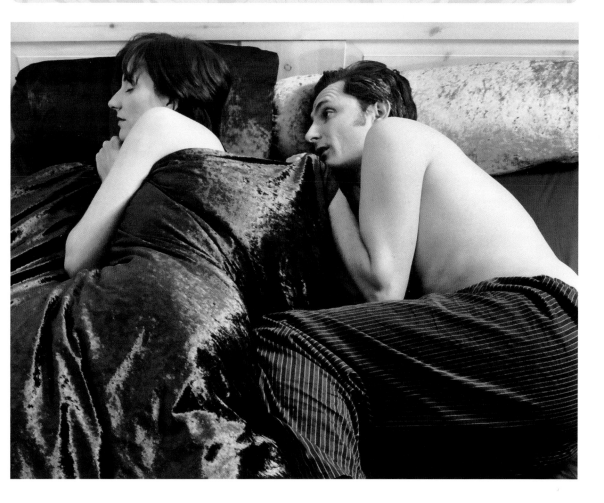

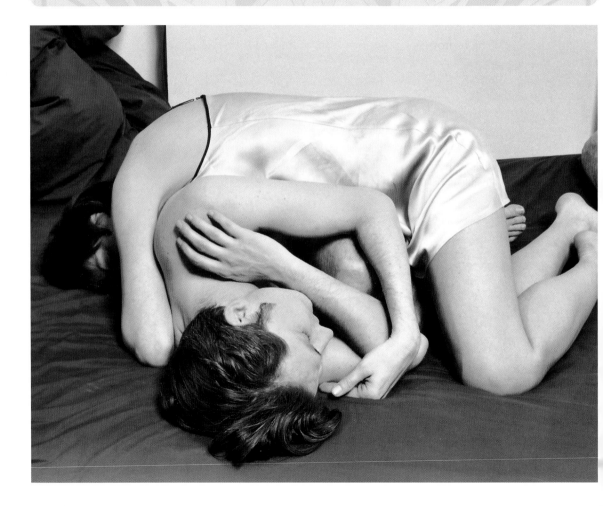

The Much Calmer Sutra shows us how comfort can be as nourishing as food.

Man Pie

Each union sees the preparation of comforts to delight, fulfil and excite the partners. *The Much Calmer Sutra* shows us how comfort can be as nourishing as food. "Man Pie" sees this allegory made flesh.

Let the more masculine of the partners assume the position of the "man." "He" should then, lying down, form a ball, acting out the part of the "filling." The other partner should now take the part of the "crust", laying themselves over the filling in the fashion of pastry.

The position is at its best enjoyed after lying for one hour under cover of a warm duvet. Massage oil may be applied for a glossy coating. For those with more culinary ambitions, the arms of the "crust" may be folded over the back in imitation of lattice-work.

No Socks, Please

Relationships require equal doses of close proximity and personal space. "No Socks, Please" offers the best of both worlds, as well as presenting a playful exercise of trust.

Let the partners lie top-to-toe on the bed, bringing the respective feet up to the area of the face. Each is now at the mercy of the other, for as the foot fears the tickle, so does the nose fear the foot.

It is vital that all parties settle upon a mutually agreed definition of acceptable personal hygiene before adopting this position. Many such unions have been ruined by inappropriately lax pedicular standards. For this reason, it is suggested that stocking and hose are rejected entirely, in favour of an "au natural" or naked foot. The ancients found liberal dustings of talcum powder a particularly efficient means of ensuring acceptable odour levels, and we may do well to follow their lead.

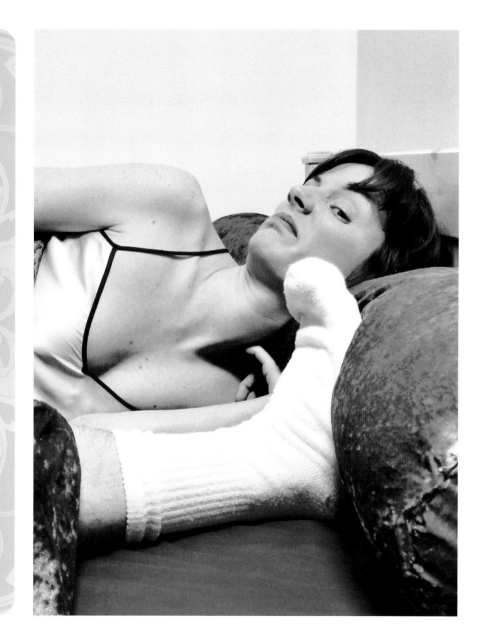

Each is

now at the

mercy of

the other,

for as the

foot fears

the tickle,

so does

the nose

fear the

foot.

Here we celebrate not only our differences,
but also our indifferences.

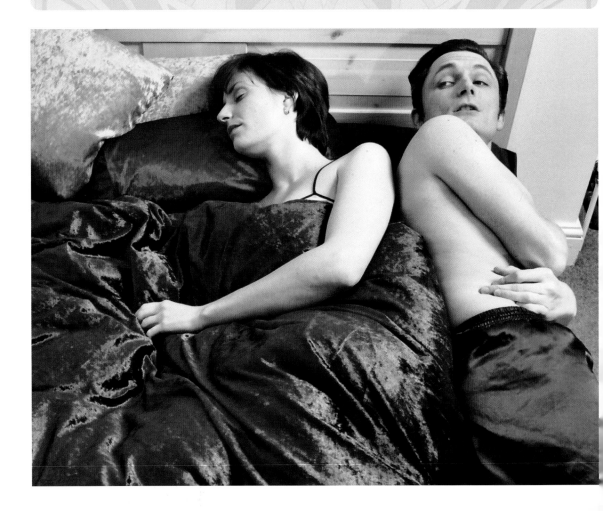

The Dog House

Relationships create responsibilities, which can in turn create blame. *The MCS* shows us the means by which lovers may outwardly express such inner feelings and, by so doing, bring them to a satisfying close. "The Dog House", while requiring communication, does not require mutual consent. One partner may decree the other to have been "dogged" without the explicit permission of the "dog." They should announce this decision without fanfare, but rather by the implied means: such as muttering; exhaling heavily; sighing; exchanging sharp glances, etc. In this way may the partner begin to guess at their canine status.

Let the partner elected "dog" return to the bed late, or in other ways have acted to the annoyance of the bedded partner, who is now called "owner". The "owner" will now dominate the bed with outstretched limbs, requiring the "dog" to enter only by means of small, subtle movements.

The "owner" shall now turn away, sighing, but in so doing contrive to further narrow the bed space available to the "dog", who is now pushed to its furthest reaches. The owner may now choose to speak, inquiring after pleasantries such as the hour of the clock or the origins of the ale-heavy fragrance of the partner. Such questions do not require a response, and any provided may invite a further narrowing of space – for the wise dog knows when to whimper.

The Poufe

"The Poufe" is, as shown, another position of apology or contrition, a means by which we may by our actions today make amends for our actions yesterday.

A karmic force runs through all relationships, a balance of responsibilities and consideration between the two parties. Any imbalance in this force, perhaps through certain acts of selfishness, may give birth to accusations, name-calling and other unpleasantness. These "forgiveness" positions serve to restore such delicate balance, offering the partner deemed to have been "wronged" the opportunity to forgive, and the other, "guilty" partner ample time to reflect on the consequences of their actions.

The guilty one will assume the position of the penitent, on knees, with hands dormant at the sides. The head will then come to rest in front of the knees, brow pressing into the surface of the bed sheet in the manner of The Thinker. Raising their legs, the other will now bring their feet to rest in an elevated position, heels resting on the lower back of the other. Both might then remain in this position until such time as the recumbent party deems this particular lesson on the importance of consideration and good deeds to have been learned.

Both might then remain in this position until such time as the recumbent party deems this particular lesson on the importance of consideration and good deeds to have been learned.

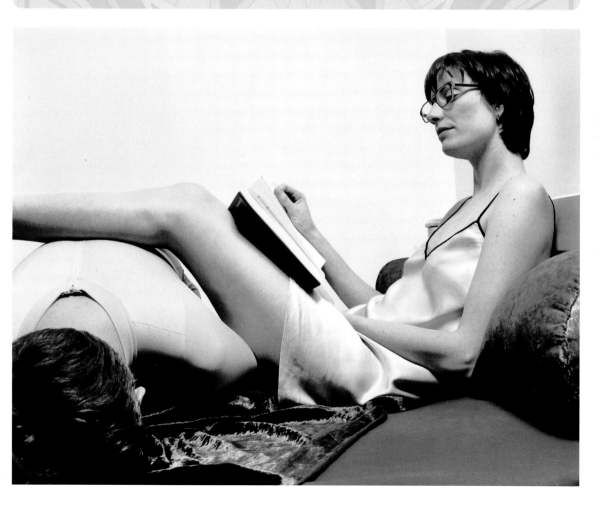

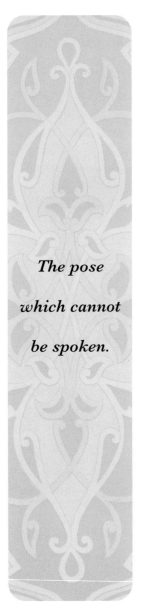

The pose

which cannot

be spoken.

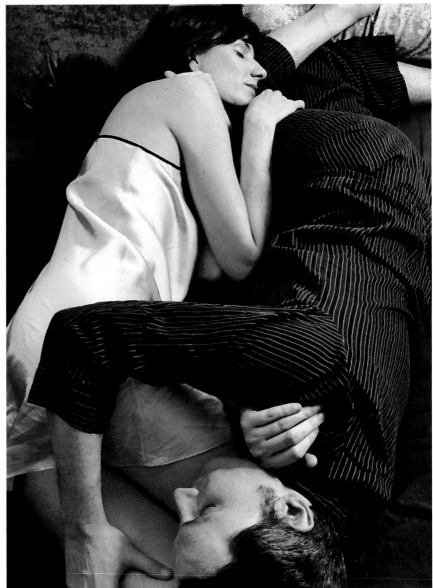

The Sound of Silence, or ''

For centuries, scholars of *The Much Calmer Sutra* have argued over the precise translation of ''. Some posit that its very unsayability makes it the most pure of all the texts, for the position that cannot be spoken is said to be the true position.

Thus the mysteries of '', known in Western countries as "The Sound Of Silence". It is presented here in a form capable of being performed in the home for the first time.

Let him lie down on his side, and inhaling the navel towards the bottom, form the shape of the numeral six, drawing his knees up towards the chest. Let her do the same, opposite, in reverse. Staring fixedly towards each the nether regions of the other, let them remain stony faced. In this manner will they come to consider the true worth of the other and in the process feel the various energies of the Universe draw to them.

Trust in such close quarters is vital, for a momentary "release" may cause disharmony and upset.

The Swallow Departs

There comes a time in a relationship when the needs of one partner do not closely match those of the other. These needs may include the desire for refreshments, for entertainment or indeed the pursuit of one of the positions described in the "Solo" section of this edition.

Such needs may be considered selfish by the more restful of the partners, who, if awakened, may wish to insist on the presence of the other or their participation in arduous physical exertions. Being caught is a painful experience and may call for a great deal of explanation and several acts of contrition. "The Swallow Departs" shows us how the exiting partner may do so in a sympathetic and silent manner.

A toe should be extended, gently, and made to touch the floor. The foot may then roll from toe to heel, touching the ground entirely. With the weight resting on this foot, the "swallow" will inch by degrees from the bed until a second and then the third limb may be lowered to the floor. He will allow the weight of the body to fall gently to the carpet, and only then will he inch towards the door. The swallow, however, must beware, for one counter for this move is the powerful and dangerous "Napping Cat" in which the apparently dormant partner reveals themselves to be awake through the airing of icy commentary.

Being caught is a painful experience and may call for a great deal of explanation and several acts of contrition.

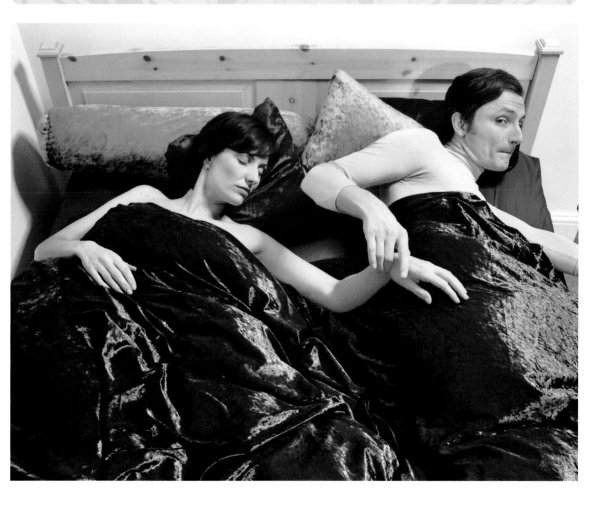

Solo

Many, on first encountering *The Much Calmer Sutra*, may see it as simply an extension of the physical life of two partners. Such a view, however, precludes those many seekers of inner calm who through choice or circumstance find themselves alone.

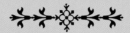

Theirs is a decision which may be challenged frequently by society or by family, and their condition can be stereotyped unfairly as that of the lonely or desperate.

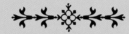

The Much Calmer Sutra, by comparison, sees singlehood not as a curse but an opportunity – a means by which intense personal pleasures may be sought out and indulged. These pleasures may include those which are too personal (or too shocking) to air with another human. Here, however, in the safety of one's own home, one can freely attempt positions of uncompromised joy. Some give hope to the distressed and some comfort to the disoriented but all fly proudly the flag of the single person, unashamed of their natural state.

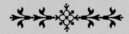

A word of caution, however – those that become used to pleasing themselves thusly may find the passage back to a relationship (should the opportunity ever arise) increasingly difficult to make. Caution must be the watchword, for these are dangerously tempting positions and only the very strong may resist the urge to succumb to them utterly…and remain happily alone.

A Toe Too Far

The more practised disciple of *The Much Calmer Sutra* is able to exert precise control over the most complex of situations with a minimum of effort.

Let the foot extended in "Dipping the Toe" extend yet even further and, with a prolonged intake of breath, let the toes curl as if fingers underneath the desired object, while simultaneously holding down the operating buttons with the pointed toe of the opposite foot. In this manner, will both feet grasp the chosen form of entertainment. Our illustration suggests a modern variant on the traditional wooden puzzles of the ancient world. Having secured such control, enjoy the gaming opportunities afforded, in accordance with the manufacturer's instructions.

A word of warning: such skill, when indulged too frequently or with too much abandon, may become an unappealing habit and this pattern may not be conducive to happy relationships, save those between a man and his leisure pursuits. This is at base a selfish position and, as our illustration shows, prowess may have served to exclude the less able partner, who is not pictured here.

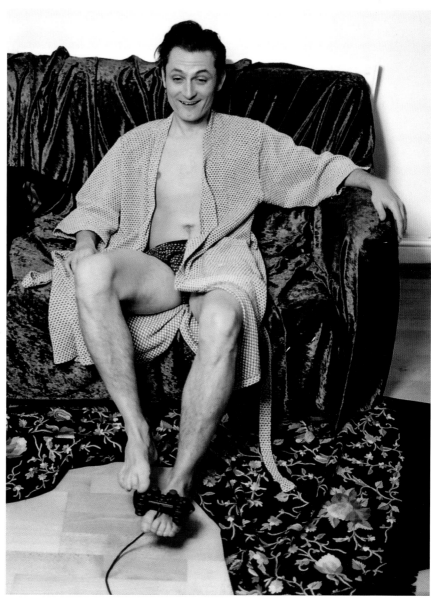

The mastery of the leisure arts does call for long, solitary nights

A healthy hand might refrain from straying below the area of the waist, for no-one would wish to be forced to reject their own advances.

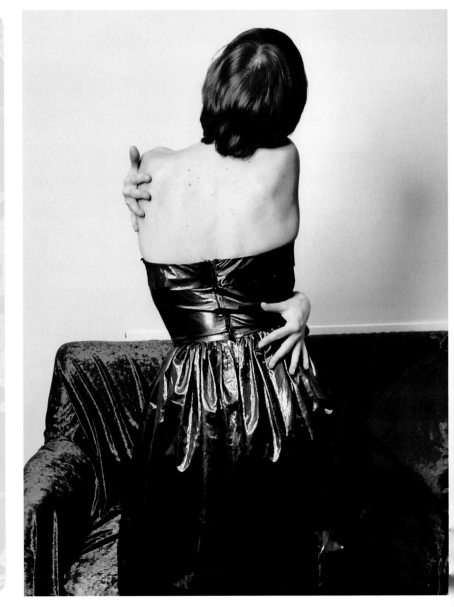

Dancing With Myself

Some "singled" persons, starved of the affection associated with relationships, may take to pleasuring themselves by their own hands.

This is of course an entirely healthy impulse and indulging it is the mark of an emotionally mature single person. Many have troubled themselves needlessly with guilt, imagining that such behaviour makes them unsuitable for relationships. Some too have suggested that the position here smacks of desperation, of a pining for human company. Rather, such movements offer the poseur a chance to delight in their own company. As more than one scholar has suggested, this affection is, perhaps, the greatest love of all.

Let the favoured music of the participant be chosen and placed upon the music device. Let them stand and, grasping the right shoulder with left hand, and right with left, begin to move in time to the sounds. As they do, let their hands wander up and down the back in search of comfort/excitement. A healthy hand might refrain from straying below the area of the waist, for no-one would wish to be forced to reject their own advances.

This position is called "Dancing With Myself" and is best suited to the latter part of a long evening which has found the "dancer" alone.

The Coffee Table

In keeping with the open, egalitarian nature of *The Much Calmer Sutra*, all positions are gender-neutral and may be performed to mutual satisfaction by either sex. However, certain positions do lend themselves more to the man or to the woman, and admitting this fact should not cause us concern.

Few know solitude as the single man knows it. Behind his locked doors may lurk such pleasures as are unfit to be aired in public. Without any eye of judgement upon him he may take to sedentary, savage ways, such as pleased our ancestors, back from the hunt and keen to conserve their energies. An indulgence along these lines may be a salutary experience for modern man, more used to pleasing others than himself. Many have found true happiness in such joyful calm.

In "The Coffee Table", man takes upon himself the responsibilities more commonly associated with household furniture, acting as a receptacle for what food or drink might cause to spill from his recumbency. He must first assume the fully prone position of the man at rest, extended to full length upon the sofa. Positioned near to hand may be such stuffs as give him pleasure – cooled beverages, snacks of potato and salt. He will reach for these without shifting body weight or angle of repose and consume them only by means of the angle of the hand – not through movement of the head or neck. A cushion may aid in this act.

Now may he sigh contentedly, and if need be, fall to sleep.

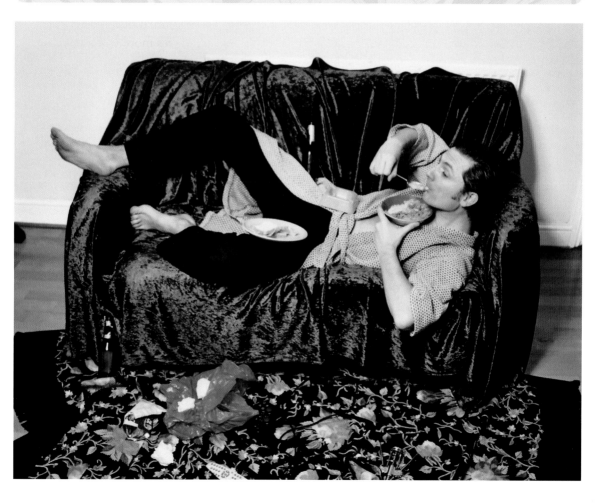

Behind his locked doors may lurk such pleasures as are unfit to be aired in public.

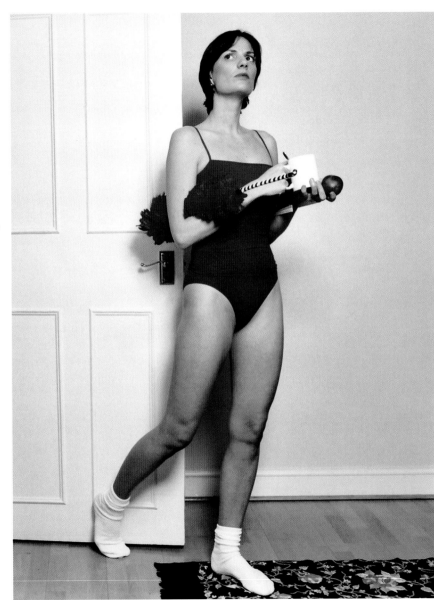

Pottering:

perhaps the

most ancient

of the

leisurely arts

The Potter

While the great drive of *The Much Calmer Sutra* is towards a shared pursuit of comfort, it has always been frankly admitted that a time may come when each must follow their own path to joy.

One such joy is that of pottering, perhaps the most ancient of the leisurely arts. The hermits of 3rd Century Egypt knew the act as "The Killer of the Noonday Demon", in tribute to the way in which an indulged potter may serve to slay the threat of ennui. "The Potter" is the literal enemy of boredom, filling "down" time instead with a series of vague pleasures of trivial import.

This position may be held for several hours at a time, and yet one called to account may be unable to speak precisely for time spent thus. Such is the great mystery of pottering, for though it fills the time, it immediately leaves the mind. This idea reaches its apex in the act of the woman shown here. She has entered the room on a mission of extremely low importance – the fetching of cutlery, for instance, or the turning on of a radio – and in the act, has wholly disremembered the motive that spurred her in the first place. She does not know why she is here, and neither do we.

The Toad in the Hole

Our comfort can easily become dependent on the whim of another.
This is particularly so in cold climates, when the winter months can be
harsh for the solitary male or female. This period of hibernation has given
birth to many seasonal unions of convenience, with warmth a driving force.

But comfort is not the sole province of the relationshipped. Many lonely
souls have found true satisfaction in the embrace of nothing more than
a simple duvet. Such happiness is held by some hermits to be the highest
form of relaxation.

No union could embrace singlehood more thoroughly, and indulgently,
than that shown here. All the consideration of the relationship is thrown
out of the window, as the body takes a chance to literally "have it all."
Gripping the edge of the quilt, the indulgent one rolls towards the other
extreme of the bed, in the process wrapping self entirely in the duvet.
They should be all but invisible to the naked eye, with only head
and toes showing from the material. In this way does the "toad" poke
from the hole, and looking about them see the true pleasures of solitude.

Many lonely souls have found true satisfaction in the embrace of nothing more than a simple duvet.

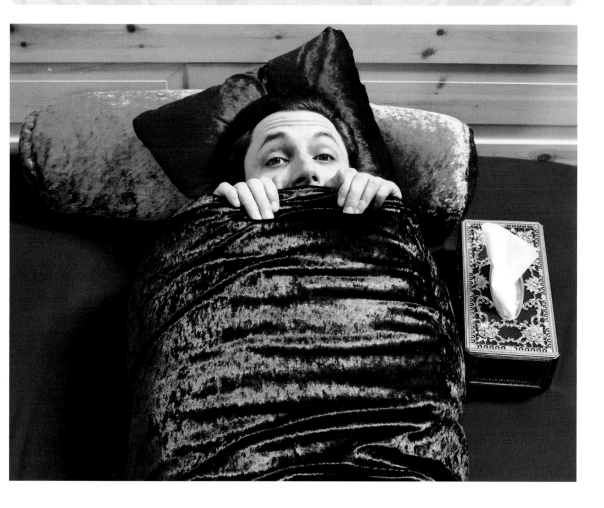

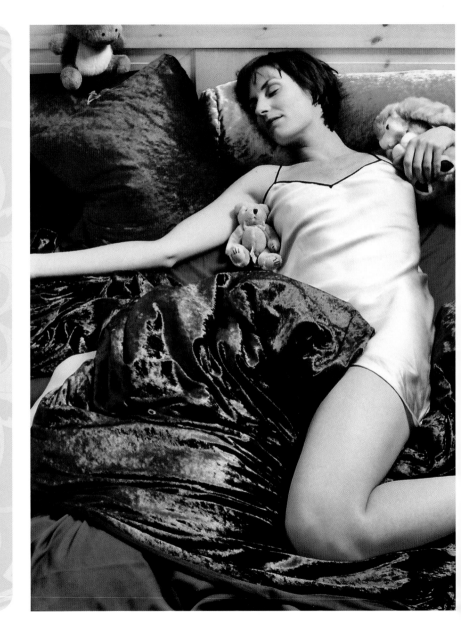

Indulging

these urges

is the only

way to deal

with them in

a healthy

and adult

manner.

The Sprawl of the Wild

Many of us become profoundly accustomed to company, and indeed *The Much Calmer Sutra* teaches us the benefits of such reliance. However, on occasion and due to no fault of our own, circumstances beyond our control may find us occupying a sleeping area alone.

Such circumstances exert a powerful influence on us, a call to answer our basest and most savage desires. Indulging these urges is the only way to deal with them in a healthy and adult manner.

"The Sprawl of the Wild" shows us one popular path to solitary pleasure. The poser is shown spreading themselves out in an apparently chaotic manner. There is method in the madness, though, as the extremities of the body are arranged in such a way that each colonise a different portion of the bed. In this manner is the bed reclaimed, "owned" again, and thus do we proclaim: I am single, and happy, for I can please myself.

Great caution should be taken to avoid taking a pillow or stuffed animal in one's hands, for such objects make poor substitutes for the pleasures of the flesh, and are considered a low form of congress indeed.

The Thinker

This position employs the relaxed sense of responsibility that comes with singlehood and is particularly suited to the "small hours" that follow an evening of revelry. The poseur sits in the normal fashion at the kitchen table or desk until such time as a need for a period of reflection presents itself. Such physical reactions are the body's way of demanding a "rest cure". This state may make itself known by a drooping of eyelids or by the apparent spinning of the room.

Our ancestors knew indulgence well and had many cures for the excess of pleasure. Above all, they saw a palliative comfort in the pressing of the head onto soothingly cool surfaces. Here the cold wood or laminate of the table allows the troubled brow to rest, whilst the upper body relaxes.

Great care should be taken to remove any foodstuffs which may happen to be nearby, lest they become affixed to the face. In the environment of the truly single person, such marks may remain for several days, for there is no-one to call out to them and say "you have kebab upon your chin".

This state may make itself known by a drooping of eyelids or by the apparent spinning of the room.

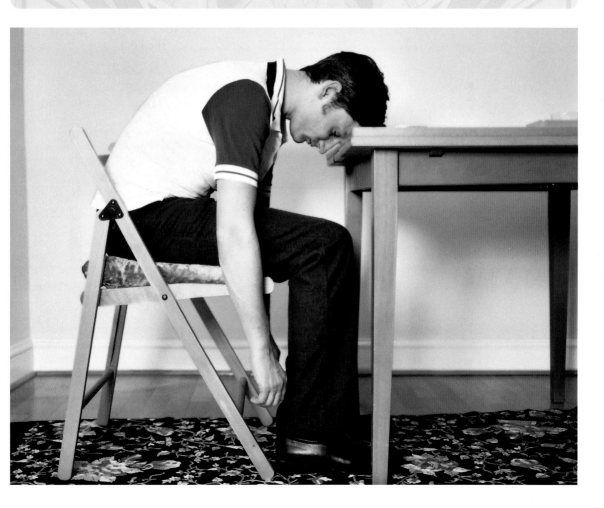

New Horizons

This book has, we hope, offered a glimpse into ancient and wondrous pleasures. Some of the positions featured may seem initially to be strange and new to us, yet all are as old as seating itself, and can generally be achieved with relatively little effort.

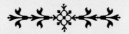

The author has been scrupulous in ensuring that all the positions pictured thus far are within the reach of the average person. None has forced the body into wholly new places, nor caused the poser any significant discomfort beyond that which might occur in the everyday course of business. We have deliberately concentrated in this selection on such easy-to-perform positions, in the hope that this guide may appeal to all and make clear that comfort is the right of everyone, regardless of physical conditioning or prowess.

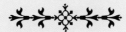

There exists, however, a series of positions which might come best under the heading "advanced." They seek to push the envelope of comfort into territories which have lain unexplored for millennia. The editors have decided to present them here in their raw, unvarnished, natural forms, in the public interest. Such matters as are described here may be unpalatable to some, shocking to others.

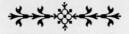

We do not judge these positions, nor take legal responsibility for any consequences which may result from their enactment. They present a world for the adventurous only, that brave breed willing to take human experience to the next level.

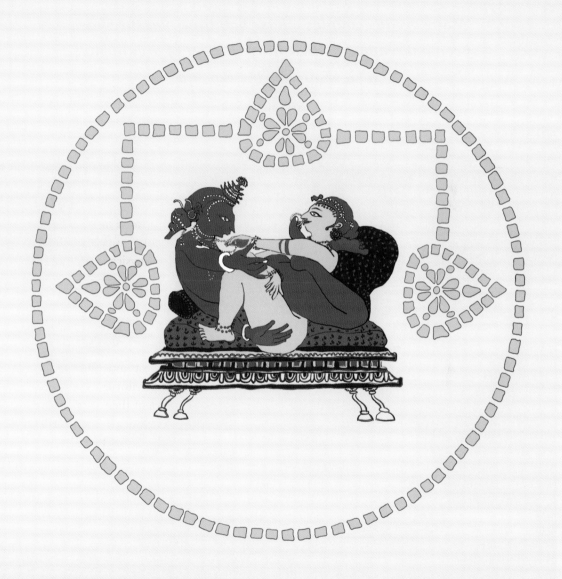

Many are the couples whose bathtime pleasure has been interrupted by that most ancient of arguments: who shall take the tap-end?

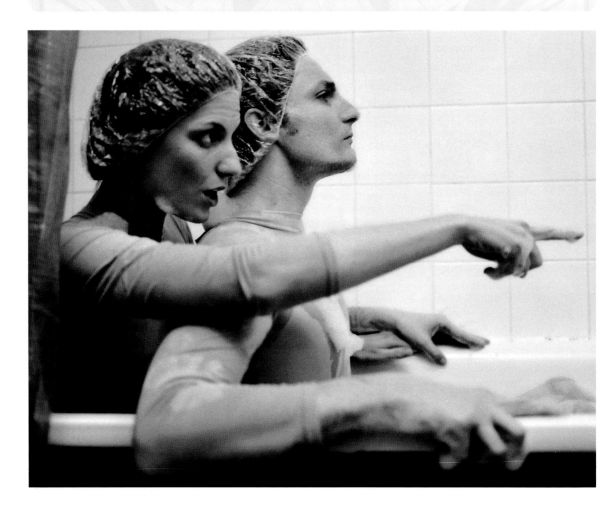

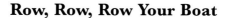

Row, Row, Row Your Boat

Many are the couples whose bathtime pleasure has been interrupted by that most ancient of arguments: who shall take the tap-end? *The Much Calmer Sutra* proposes various solutions to this eternal conundrum but none are as satisfying as this.

In the position, the couple ensure an equal distribution of comfort by positioning themselves away from the tap end. He or she reclines in the bath, having applied such unguents and soaps as deemed necessary. The presence of rubber matting may aid in ensuring that they remain fixed in position.

Sighing, the seater must then part both legs and allow the partner to step in, settling into a seated position in between the proffered legs so that both now face the taps. Arms may be outstretched to grip the sides of the bath, or imaginary oars, as both deem fit.

Great fun may now be had in simulating the experience of a rowing boat, with each partner taking it in turns to "cox" the other with shouted instructions regarding their movements, the soap, etc.

Splash

Common sense and inherited memory tells us that water is a precious commodity and that to waste it is a sin.

Such thinking, while eminently sensible, is diametrically opposed to the pleasure-seeking principles that underpin *The Much Calmer Sutra*. Rather, we advocate here a sensual abandon.

Let each bather lay down towels and other coverings over such surfaces which may not benefit from wetness. Let the tub be filled to brimming, and such foams, soaps and oils be added as appropriate.

Upon completion of the running of the tub, they should both attempt to gain entry, competing as if this were a race. The force of their entry will be marked by the degree to which water is displaced and much satisfaction may be had with this action.

The first in the tub may celebrate with further splashing, which may in turn beget splashing. This should continue until the displaced water outside is of greater quantity to that which is in the tub, or until either partner is comprehensively wet.

A heedless delight in the wonders of water.

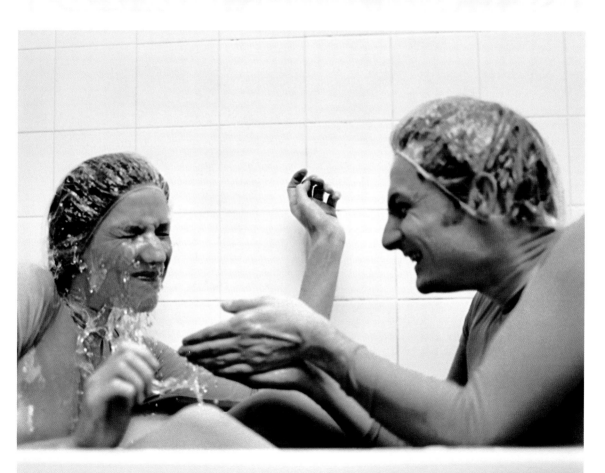

Relishing this power, she may choose not to give it up without reward.

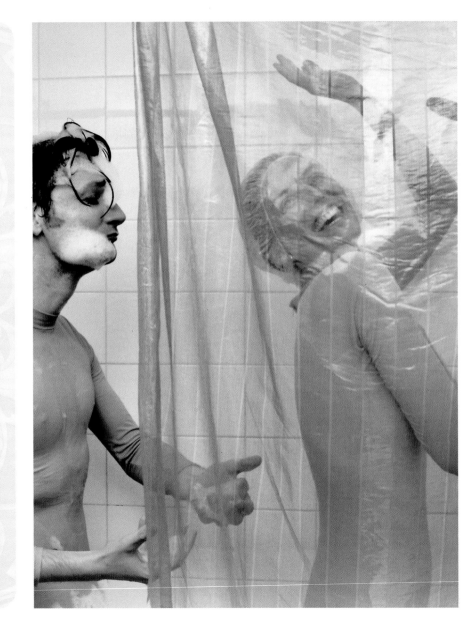

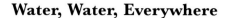

Water, Water, Everywhere

Nowhere is the importance of a considered and selfless sharing of resources more keenly felt than in the bathroom, where towels, soaps and even water itself may be the subject of quarrels. Here we must learn to practise supreme patience in understanding the needs of the loved one and must refrain from accusations of time-wasting or indulgence as well as the calling out of questions, such as "what are you *doing* in there?"

"Water, Water, Everywhere" shows us one such contested situation and suggests the means to resolve it.

Both partners have entered the showering area together, yet there is only one stream of water. They must, then, take turns to enjoy such hot water as is available. Stepping to the rear, he has begun to shampoo himself in anticipation of the availability of rinsing. She, however, has turned her back to him, luxuriating in the excess of liquid. Relishing this power, she may choose not to give it up without reward.

He will then entreat her, begging, and ask that he be permitted a small amount of water and will point to his chattering teeth and soap-blinded eyes as evidence of this deep need. She may be unimpressed and focus on a task at hand, such as the removal of unwanted hair from the leg. Only when his entreaties reach such pitch as necessary for her heart to become softened will she consider offering him the shower.

The Sleeping Mule

Many couples, having spent some considerable time together, may find the pleasures of the bedroom beginning to pall. The playing of games is one way to re-establish that sense of fun we may find in each other.

"The Sleeping Mule" is based on a childhood game popular in sixth century Arabia. This was a culture which had only recently discovered the process of fermentation, and courtiers flush with jars of "ale" were keen for entertainment to match their playful moods. Thus was a game for children adapted for the courts of the sultan. There, princes would goad each other into the consumption of massive qualities of "golden shame", until such time as one or the other passed into unconsciousness. Seeing his incapacity, his friends might then spring upon him and, taking whatever materials were to hand, seek to decorate him comically, and rest objects upon the sleeping form. Having ridiculed him thus, they would call for an artist and command that the scene be recorded. Copies would then be circulated, to the great amusement of the court.

Lovers, of course, were quick to adapt such fun to their own ends. Here, the awakened one amuses themselves upon the prostrate form, placing objects upon the body until discovered. Daring greater and greater risks, they might culminate in the placing of an item such as a glass of water, which might then at the time of awakening be caused to spill to the great delight of the one and the puzzlement of the other.

Many couples, having spent some considerable time together,
may find the pleasures of the bedroom beginning to pall.

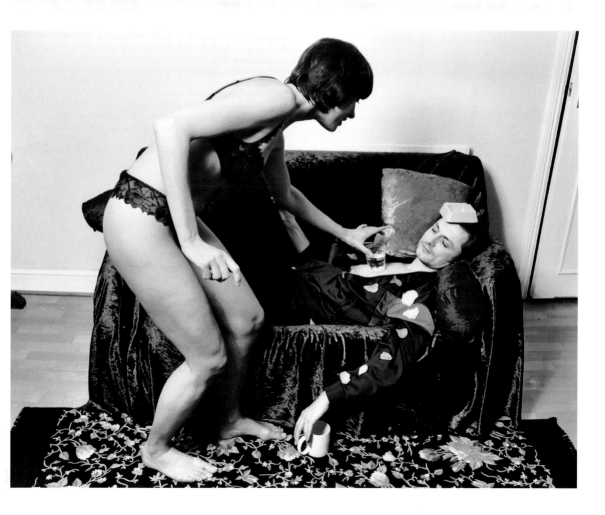

It is not unusual, though, for one partner to be more keen on such brave naturism than the other.

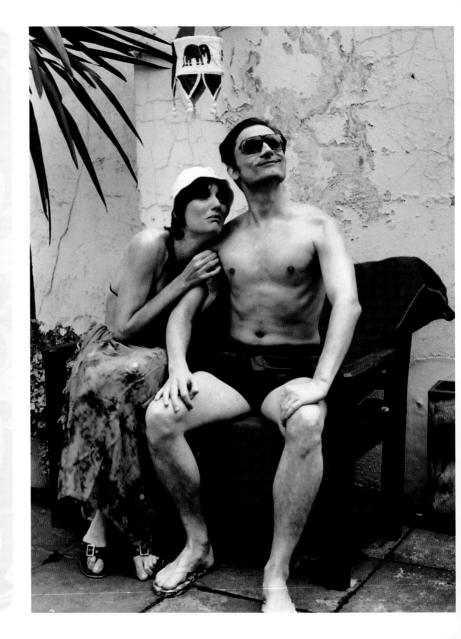

British Summer Time

Travel has broadened the modern mind, bringing new ways of relaxing learned on foreign shores and in warmer climes. This internationalism brings breadth and depth to the communal comforts we share but the opulent indulgence that such warmth offers can leave us unprepared for the demands posed by our own immediate surroundings.

The disadvantages of the less welcoming climate, however, are compensated for by the crafts of comfort which such nations offer – comforts designed to compensate for the privations imposed by Nature. We may not have sun, say the people of the North – but we have satisfying lard-based foodstuffs and seating particularly designed to reward the tired person.

This position may be enjoyed in the gardens of the home or public spaces, such as the public parks of large cities. It is at its best, however, when both are exposed to the full force of the elements on an area of land adjacent to a large body of water. Here any discomfort that gusts of wind may cause actively encourages each to find shelter in the other's arms. It is not unusual, though, for one partner to be more keen on such brave naturism than the other.

Public Convenience

The comforts described in these pages are principally those that can be
achieved in private, at home. But such privacy is a luxury in our hectic
world. Nowadays couples must snatch time together whenever they can.

Fortunately for us, our ancestors also knew such privations and devised
pleasures that might be enjoyed in precious moments, even under the eyes of
strangers. The poses they created for ancient doorways and primitive public
transport showed low-impact means of sharing physical space creatively.
Excitingly, such positions can be recreated easily in today's
space-and-time-starved world.

"Public Convenience" can be enjoyed on any form of transport,
or during a lull at an unsuccessful dinner party. It is a form of relaxation
almost invisible in its stealth and to the casual observer may be taken as
simple affection. In fact it is much more. It is each partner using the other as
a literal prop, allowing both to relax and yet remain upright.

Each sits, facing forward, adjacent to the other. Bending from the waist,
the nearest shoulders are allowed to touch gently. Leaning further in they
now fully support each other's weight. If the position is used after a meal
at the house of a neighbour, great care must be taken to guard against
the lolling of the head.

*"Public Convenience" can be enjoyed on any form of transport,
or during a lull at an unsuccessful dinner party.*

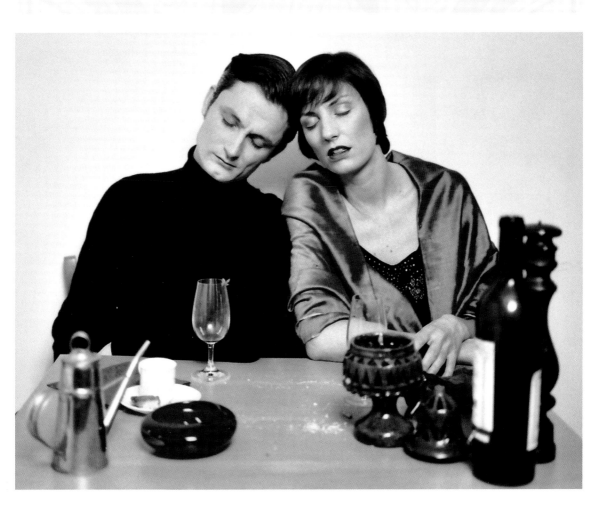

Equally, this shall be of great use to the budget travellers seeking to maximise the standard hotel bed.

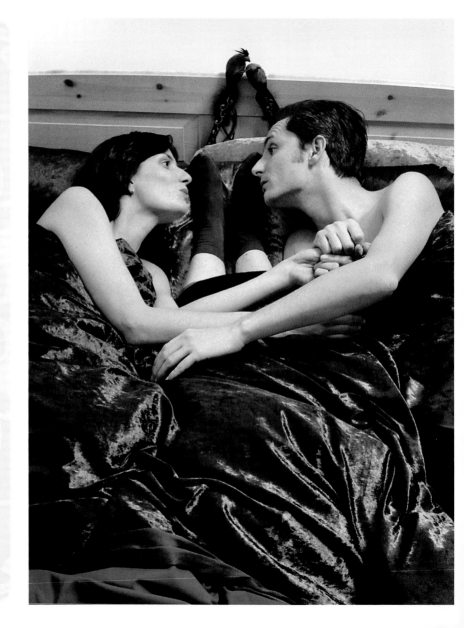

Sardines

Our ancestors saw solitude as a luxury, an indulgence to be savoured through the positions in this book. But in addition to poses suitable for such relative privacy, they sought to find ways of attaining comfort whilst coping with many persons, all eager for space. Their experience in accommodating many others simultaneously can be of great relevance to the modern city-dweller, struggling in cramped accommodations. Creative solutions are vital in comfort emergencies, such as the unplanned and lengthy social calls of acquaintances and the absence of adequate bedding.

"Sardines" artfully converts the standard double bed into accommodation for up to eight forms. Each must play their part with care, for the greater good of this bed society rests on individual responsibility. The twitcher, the kicker and the provider of noxious fumes are not welcome here.

Beginning with the furthest reaches of the bed, a person may lie prone. The next person shall take up the identical position, but in reverse, with feet facing face and vice versa. This shall be repeated, until the bed shall be entirely full, with each at pains to take up no more than their allotted space. The pedicular hygiene referred to in "No Socks, Please" should be scrupulously followed.

The Pretzel

The Much Calmer Sutra is an open, egalitarian work. Where other guides may demand a high level of physical fitness and a determined commitment to pushing the fleshy envelope, *The MCS* demands little more than a vague interest and the will to pursue comfort.

There exist, however, more complex and demanding positions and the dedicated seeker of calm, keen to move to "the next level", may wish to pursue such challenges. "The Pretzel" is one such position – offering both partners the opportunity to exploit physical flexibility towards greater and greater comfort.

Great care should be taken in assuming this position and the editors remind the reader that no legal responsibility will be assumed by them in the event of spraining, chafing or other physical injury which may result from pursuit of this suggestion.

By wrapping around each other in the manner of the breaded knot, we see physical confirmation of the entwining of our spirits. With each movement we should be mindful of the method with which it was achieved, in the manner of an explorer who may wish to retrace his steps later. For some couples have found themselves in great difficulty and have cried out for support in disentangling each from the loving embrace of the other. The fire departments of our modern age have little sympathy for such self-inflicted injury. Lubricants are considered advisable.

The fire departments of our modern age have little sympathy for such self-inflicted injury.

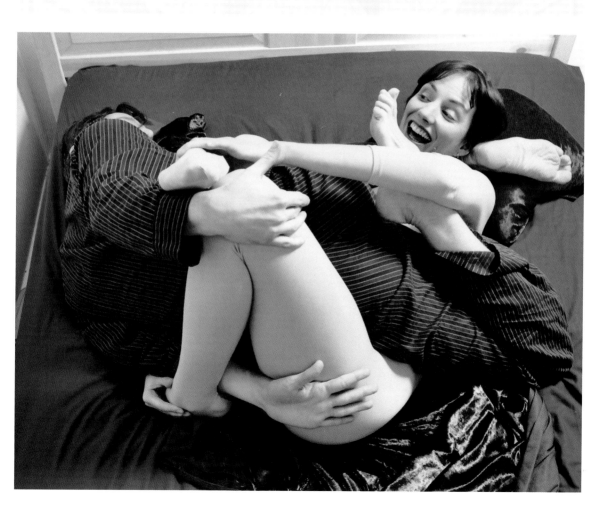

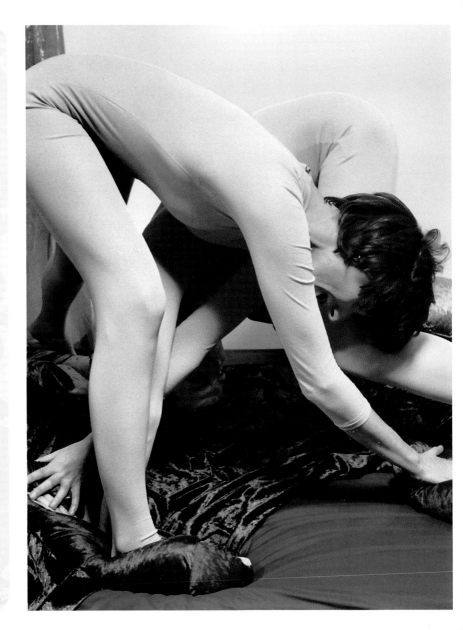

As an

icebreaker

in new

relationships

it is

invaluable.

Left Foot, Blue Pillow

"Left Foot, Blue Pillow" is a game of fun and skill for all ages, which may be played with two, three, or even four parties, dependent on the needs and proclivities of the partners. As an icebreaker in new relationships it is invaluable.

Our forbears believed in the power of chance as a positive force, best expressed through such means as the I Ching, through which apparently random elements may combine to offer insight into ourselves.

Each lies together in an agreeable starting position and nominates one partner to begin, based on whatever means seems fair, such as the person who has most recently avoided duties in the house. They will then begin to count down from five to one at an agreed rate and, on reaching one, will shout out – he a part of the bed and she a part of the body. He must then perform the act of touching said part of the bed with the part described. On her turn the same shall happen and she shall perform a similar act as nominated. In this manner each will take turns to dare the other to greater and greater physical extremes. Only when one may not perform the act, or shall cry out surrender, shall the game be declared to have been won and a victor declared. This victor may demand as their reward any trophy they deem fit, such as a position of supplication like "The Poufe" or the fetching of hot drinks and the like.

Easy Like Sunday Morning

Ancient India was a place of indulged leisure for the upper classes, a world in which a man might be judged by his ability to enjoy multiple pleasures at the same time. A young princeling might, for instance, dedicate himself to savouring a gargantuan feast whilst simultaneously enjoying games of skill and chance *and* the entertainments offered by sensual dancers, all the while contriving not to spill a drop of nectar from his bejewelled cup.

This sustained juggling of tasks is an art now wasted on the business world, where the ability to handle a telephone call, electronic mail and textual message simultaneously is the mark of a productive worker. With this position, such productivity, such skills of balance, are marshalled towards a higher and more noble goal – that of mutual comfort.

Take an assortment of articles as appropriate to the day and hour and strew them about the bed. Let each partner assume a position mid-way betwixt lying and sitting, propped and bolstered from behind by feathered cushions. Now the partners may claim ownership of that before them, taking in their hands this, and that, until all objects and foodstuffs are accounted for. The winner is not necessarily the one with the most objects but he or she with the objects which he can still eat or otherwise enjoy. Although the more practised may be able to control as many as six or seven items simultaneously, the beginner may wish to limit themselves to three items.

Here the goals of multiple pleasures and mutual satisfaction are reclaimed for leisure use.

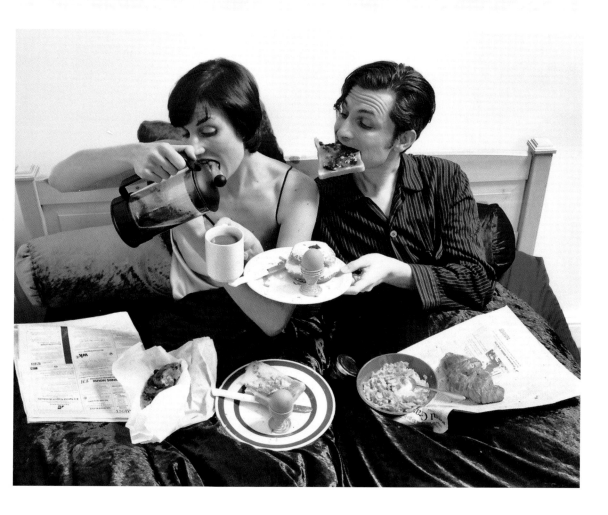

Dedication:
To Francesca, who *never* steals the quilt.

First published in 2005 by New Holland Publishers
(UK) Ltd
London • Cape Town • Sydney • Auckland
www.newhollandpublishers.com

Garfield House
86-88 Edgware Road
London W2 2EA
United Kingdom

80 McKenzie Street
Cape Town 8001
South Africa

Level 1, Unit 4
14 Aquatic Drive
Frenchs Forest
NSW 2086
Australia

218 Lake Road
Northcote
Auckland
New Zealand

10 9 8 7 6 5 4 3 2 1

ISBN 1 84537 239 5

Editorial direction: Rosemary Wilkinson
Production: Hazel Kirkman
Designer: Paul Wright
Photographer: J J Stratford
Illustrations: Byju Sukumaran

Reproduction by Modern Age, Hong Kong
Printed and bound by Craft Print International,
Singapore

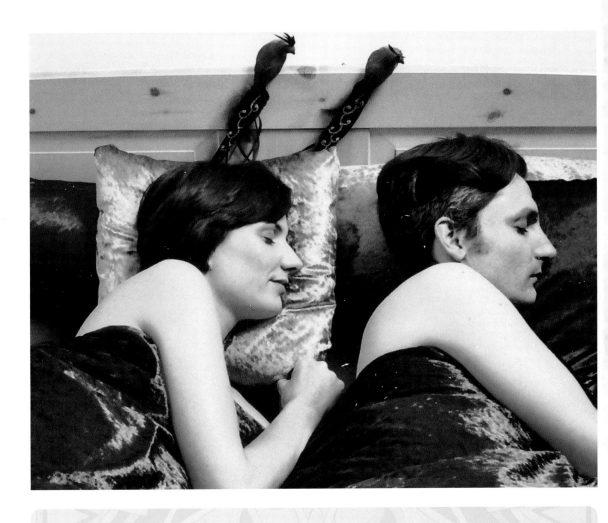

Nirvana

Acknowledgements
The author would like to express his heartfelt thanks
to his patient and flexible models, Miss High Leg
Kick (Comic Visionary Superstar,
www.misshighlegkick.com) and Name Withheld,
who should cut down on the pies. Very-special
thanks to justifiably World Famous Photo Reporter
JJ Stratford (www.jjstratford.com) and Illustrator-
about-town Byju Sukumaran. Extra-special thanks
to Editor Extraordinaire Rosemary Wilkinson,
without whose imagination and support this would
not exist and to Creative Designer, Paul Wright, who
put the words and pictures together so graphically.

The author thanks his family (especially his Mum)
and the Bagliones for their support and kindness.
Shout-outs are also due to Geraldine, Lalo,
G. Wright of www.dexys.org, Pops, Dale, Will,
The Action Men, Amber, Elan, Jem, Claire and
everyoneelsewhoknowsme.

Francesca Baglione can never be thanked enough.

To all the above, and to all readers now and in
future, he offers his most sincere apologies.